Well90

Wellness Companion

Author:

   Jeremy Stueven, M.D.

Published by Doctor of Living, LLC.

Cover art: Doctor of Living™
Visit our website at www.DoctorOfLiving.com

Introduction

Welcome to the Doctor of Living's Well90 Program™. Congratulations on your commitment to achieving wellness!

The Well90 Program™ is designed to put you on track for wellness in 90 days or less. In contrast to other health programs, our program is sustainable and built to help you achieve your health goals. In doing so, we open the pathway to true wellness, which isn't just physical, but mental and spiritual. Wellness is NOT just the absence of disease. Wellness is one's greatest potential level of functioning.

Wellness has been barred in controversy over the years, considered pseudoscience by critics, at different times in its history. The pioneers of wellness knew it's value without the evidence to support it and operated on instinct. Today, we have substantial evidence that backs our claims.

Everything you learn in this program is 100% evidence-based and backed by scientific research. What you learn in this program isn't our angle on health, it's facts. This is important, because too often health and wellness claims are not based on fact.

Our model is also 100% sustainable. It will make you feel happier, become more energetic, and become more pleased with the way you look.

We use a unique approach to wellness. Our approach looks at 5 Pillars of Health™: nutrition, physical activity, toxin avoidance, emotional wellness and spiritual connections.

Our wellness improvement process is based on engineering principles. You will first conduct a wellness assessment, then receive a custom report and consultation which will lead to a wellness plan. You will work the plan for 90 days, using our wellness companion: a workbook or guide. Then, you will be re-assessed with our program. This whole process is known as the wellness improvement process.

We are complex mental, physical and spiritual beings. Medicine has reduced us to machines over the last 100 years, which has helped in diagnosis and treatment of disease, which has led to disintegration of the of the understanding of our whole. Wellness requires an approach that considers the whole person.

Wellness is a term that has been overused and even misused, but comes out of a school of medical thought, originally envisioned by Dr. Halbert Dunn. He was the "father of the wellness movement."

Dr. Dunn looked at good health as "not being ill" but rather as having "high-level wellness" a "condition of change in which the individual moves forward, climbing toward a higher potential of functioning." This led to the holistic health movement, furthered by Drs. Don Ardell, Robert Russell, John Travis and Elizabeth Neilson.

At Doctor of Living, we have adopted this model of wellness. We seek nothing less than your highest level of functioning. We will use data to create a custom wellness plan for wellness improvement. We will study the changes over 90 days. Finally, we will create a sustainable life plan that you can continue to use.

Wellness is not a substitute for primary care. We will not diagnose, treat or attempt to treat any ailment, disease or condition.

Doctor of Living is as much a new philosophy on wellness, as it is a movement. I am glad that you are now part of this movement. I know that you find this model to be helpful and sustainable. Thanks for taking me on your wellness journey. Let's get started!

As questions come up, please email as at contact@doctorofliving.com.

Thanks for joining us…let's learn and grow,

Dr. Jeremy

Table of Contents

Meal Planning Introduction

The food we eat creates energy for every cell in our body, which we need to survive. In addition, food provides nutrients and vitamins that help our minds and bodies to thrive. Food carries the potential, in many cases, to heal our bodies. On the contrary, food can create too much energy for our bodies, expose us to toxins, inflame our bodies and cause disease. We usually think of food from the perspective of energy and pleasure, but rarely do we consider all the above with every meal.

Planning the food we eat each week in advance, helps us to ensure that food is nutritious and not harmful. Spontaneous meals are unlikely to meet all our body's needs, so pre-planning meals is essential to achieving health and wellness through food. There are many ways that you can create a convenient home-cooked meal, served at home or away. We will help you plan the meal, come up with your shopping list and make it happen!

First, pick a day of the week when you like to shop. You should do your meal planning before shopping. For example, if you plan on shopping on Saturday afternoon, then plan your meals on Saturday morning or Friday evening. We have recommended several meals on our website from cookbooks that we have purchased and love. Each of the meals within the cookbooks will have a complete list of ingredients.

At first, you may need to stock up on a few things that are new and different. It may be a little more expensive at first, but over time you will begin to have more of the ingredients these recipes are calling for.

Select meals not just for dinner, but for all meals. Select snacks and place them on the plan. This makes you accountable and ensures that you have anticipated being hungry and needing snacks. Needing a snack is nothing to feel guilty about. Eating snacks is important and necessary. The good news is that on a plant-based diet, you can eat a few healthy snacks and be just fine.

We never count calories in the Well 90 Program™. I know that it's tempting, but it's a major source of anxiety and frustration for most and completely unnecessary for all. Meals that are plant-based, healthy snacks, avoiding animal protein, and avoiding sugar means that you are unlikely to be eating too many calories. Counting calories only leads to starving oneself, which is not sustainable and reduces your intake of nutritious foods necessary for health. Calories, themselves, are necessary for human life.

Let's get started:

1. Grab a pencil, just in case you need to change something.
2. Open our list of cookbooks/potential meals.
3. Place the name of the desired meal for each time-period in the respective column for each day with snack information.
4. Look at the checkbox on the right for each day. This gives you goals for each day. It may not be possible to get 100%, but the closer you get to daily goals, the closer you get to health. Shoot for 100%!
5. Check the boxes BEFORE you finish the day. If you don't have what you need on the checkbox, you can eras and revise things.
6. Place a stickie on each page of the cookbooks as you are writing the names down for each day.
7. Once you have written each down and checked the boxes for the day, now write out the recipe ingredients into your shopping list. We have specifically placed the shopping list on a separate page. For some people, it might be easiest to rip this page out and bring it along to the store. For others, you may want to bring the whole manual. Another popular way to do it, is to take a quick picture and then open your phone at the store and look at what you have written out. Whatever works best, but never try and guess. You will buy too much, the wrong stuff or not enough. Staying honest to your plan is part of the process and very important.

At the end of each week, take some notes. Comment on what worked and what didn't. Reflect on what you might tweak from the recipe.

Physical Activity Instructions

CAUTION: *You should discuss all physical activity with your physician prior to engaging in any activity. Failure to do so, ramping up to quickly or pushing yourself beyond your safety zone could cause harm.*

Physical activity isn't just about exercise. Exercise is a word that many of us dread. It is incredibly important, but there is more to physical activity than just exercise.

Our sleep patterns fall into physical activity. Rest and restoration is necessary for healing. Generally obtaining 7-8 hours of nightly sleep should be your target. Too much sleep > 8 hours is just as harmful as not enough < 7 hours.

Weights are necessary to maintaining strength, not just for how you look, but for long-term conditioning, body stability, and balance. Shoot for at least 120 minutes per week to start with.

Movement opposes being sedentary. Sedentariness is more associated with the occurrence of disease than exercise is with the avoidance of disease. In other words, movement is of the utmost importance. This is where the number of steps daily comes into discussion. Your goal, at some point should be 10,000 steps daily, but start comfortable and work towards this goal.

Aerobic exercise is important to avoiding disease and isn't the same as your number of steps. You should plan an activity that you enjoy. Running isn't for everyone and gym machines don't work for everyone either. Choose an activity that you enjoy. Your goal should be 150 minutes per week.

Stretching is an activity that I find to be helpful every day. The best way to do this is buy a yoga mat and to learn some basic Yoga techniques. These techniques can help to avoid injury, build balance and build strength.

Nature Observation Instructions

Getting out outside for 30-60 minutes daily is important to overall wellness. There is a sense of awe by the beauty created by our Creator. There have been numerous studies about health improvement and in being in nature. In fact, there is one such study that looked at the oscillations of the Earth (the Earth is always moving) and these oscillations create euphoria with people. Euphoria is a sense of well-being and peace.

While you are outside and in nature, you should reflect on the following themes this week.

Beauty-Beauty is in the eye of the beholder. Nothing is beautiful to everyone. Search your soul and find those things in nature that are beautiful to you. From animals, to insects, to butterflies, the sky above or moving water. Whatever you see that moves you, reflect on it. Write it down. Draw a brief picture or sketch. Engage with it in a way that is meaningful. The beauty of what you see is a gift from our Creator. Your eyes, your reflections. Focus on those ideas and immerse yourself in beauty.

Feel/Touch-When you are in nature there are many things to feel (physically) and touch. Do you feel the wind against your face? Do you feel warmth from the sun? Do you feel a bit from the cold? Go ahead and touch something around you. Touch some soft moss growing on a rock. Touch a leaf. Touch a flower. Touch the rough bark on a tree. Touch mud. Touch a cool rock. How do you feel when you touch? Many times, we are told "don't touch that," but in nature, it's ok to touch most things. Obviously, use caution with certain common sense items. Touch and physical feeling are important to reflect on.

Hearing-What do you hear when you close your eyes? Do you hear birds? Do you hear wind? Do you hear children playing? Do you hear insects? What about moving water? These are the sounds of or music of nature. As you immerse yourself within the sounds, keep your eyes close for several minutes and reflect on it.

Spiritual Letters Instructions

This is an optional activity, as some people may feel uncomfortable with the Divine/God. It is our belief at Doctor of Living that our spiritual health determines our emotional and physical health. Our spirituality is the basis by which our health is created, how we see and interact with the world. Over the next 12 weeks, we would like you to work on the following topics. Some of them will be directly to God and others associated more with inter-relationships. We will provide worksheets to help you do so.

Instructions:
This workbook is designed for you and you alone. You are free to share with trusted others, but you should plan to keep most of it to yourself, as your answers and thoughts will likely be more genuine.

Each week, you will have a new spiritual devotion to reflect upon. You will be challenged to write a letter to God. We want you to have the weekends for rest and reflection. It would be helpful to jot down your thoughts about the topic. Try to jot down what comes to mind first, without editing. We will explore your past, present and future. As you do so, you may experience joy and comfort, pain and remorse, or even fear. It is natural to feel these emotions. Just as when you meditate, try to experience these emotions without any judgment. You are not alone in having many emotions about your spiritual well-being.

16

Gratitude Journal Instructions

The gratitude journal should be a time to reflect on the things that make you happy, things you are grateful for, times where you noticed something nice. The purpose of this exercise is to pause and appreciate. Take some time each week to journal about the things that made you smile, made you laugh, showed unexpected kindness, or made you happy.

Art/Beauty Journaling Instructions

The purpose of the Art/Beauty journaling is to take the time to appreciate beautiful things in your life. Each week you should spend some time enjoying art, music or another form of beauty that inspires you. The journal is to allow you to write down your thoughts or draw the beautiful things you experienced. Each week we have given you a prompt if you would like to use it. Otherwise, feel free to journal on whatever inspires you.

Weekly Activity Logs

Week 1

1) Meal Planning/Log
- ☐ Write recipe name (and cookbook and page number)
- ☐ Check goals against meal plan for the day
- ☐ Create grocery list
- ☐ Make changes to meals if altered so log is accurate

2) Physical Activity
- ☐ Jot hours of sleep night before and any notes
- ☐ Document weight training (if applicable)
- ☐ Document aerobic exercise
- ☐ Complete stretching
- ☐ Record steps at end of day

3) Complete Toxin Avoidance activity
- ☐ See customized wellness plan for recommended activity

4) Complete Emotional Wellness activity
- ☐ Meditate daily
- ☐ Follow emotional wellness plan

5) (Optional) Write Spiritual Letter
- ☐ Complete a spiritual letter theme

6) Nature Journal
- ☐ Commit to 30 mins/day outside. Use the journal to jot your thoughts/drawings for the week.

7) Art/Beauty/Music Appreciation
- ☐ Incorporate fresh flowers into your home this week.

Week 1 – Meal Planning

	Breakfast	Lunch	Dinner	Snacks	Goals
Monday					☐ 2 fruit ☐ 1 berry ☐ 5 veggies ☐ 1 cruciferous ☐ 1 leafy green ☐ Legume ☐ Whole grain ☐ Flax/Chia ☐ Nut/Seed
Tuesday					☐ 2 fruit ☐ 1 berry ☐ 5 veggies ☐ 1 cruciferous ☐ 1 leafy green ☐ Legume ☐ Whole grain ☐ Flax/Chia ☐ Nut/Seed
Wednesday					☐ 2 fruit ☐ 1 berry ☐ 5 veggies ☐ 1 cruciferous ☐ 1 leafy green ☐ Legume ☐ Whole grain ☐ Flax/Chia ☐ Nut/Seed
Thursday					☐ 2 fruit ☐ 1 berry ☐ 5 veggies ☐ 1 cruciferous ☐ 1 leafy green ☐ Legume ☐ Whole grain ☐ Flax/Chia ☐ Nut/Seed

	Breakfast	Lunch	Dinner	Snacks	Goals
Friday					☐ 2 fruit ☐ 1 berry ☐ 5 veggies ☐ 1 cruciferous ☐ 1 leafy green ☐ Legume ☐ Whole grain ☐ Flax/Chia ☐ Nut/Seeds
Saturday					☐ 2 fruit ☐ 1 berry ☐ 5 veggies ☐ 1 cruciferous ☐ 1 leafy green ☐ Legume ☐ Whole grain ☐ Flax/Chia ☐ Nut/Seeds
Sunday					☐ 2 fruit ☐ 1 berry ☐ 5 veggies ☐ 1 cruciferous ☐ 1 leafy green ☐ Legume ☐ Whole grain ☐ Flax/Chia ☐ Nut/Seeds

Notes:

_____

_____

_____

Week 1 - Physical Activity

	Sleep	Weights/ Resistance	Steps	Aerobic Exercise	Stretching
Monday					
Tuesday					
Wednesday					
Thursday					
Goals	7-8 Hours	120 min/week (30 min/day three-four times/week)	10,000 steps daily	150 minutes /week	20 minutes /day

	Sleep	Weights/ Resistance	Steps	Aerobic Exercise	Stretching
Friday					
Saturday					
Sunday					
Goals	7-8 Hours	120 min/week (30 min/day three-four times/week)	10,000 steps daily	150 minutes /week	20 minutes /day

Notes

_____
_____
_____
_____
_____

Nature Journal
Week 1

Gratitude Journal

_____

_____

_____

_____

_____

Meditation

☐ Sunday   ☐ Thursday

☐ Monday   ☐ Friday

☐ Tuesday   ☐ Saturday

☐ Wednesday

Additional Notes

_____

_____

_____

_____

_____

_____

_____

_____

_____

Week 2

1) Meal Planning/Log
- ☐ Write recipe name (and cookbook and page number)
- ☐ Check goals against meal plan for the day
- ☐ Create grocery list
- ☐ Make changes to meals if altered so log is accurate

2) Physical Activity
- ☐ Jot hours of sleep night before and any notes
- ☐ Document weight training (if applicable)
- ☐ Document aerobic exercise
- ☐ Complete stretching
- ☐ Record steps at end of day

3) Complete Toxin Avoidance activity
- ☐ See customized wellness plan for recommended activity

4) Complete Emotional Wellness activity
- ☐ Meditate daily
- ☐ Follow emotional wellness plan

5) (Optional) Write Spiritual Letter
- ☐ Complete a spiritual letter theme

6) Nature Journal
- ☐ Commit to 30 mins/day outside. Use the journal to jot your thoughts/drawings for the week.

7) Art/Beauty/Music Appreciation
- ☐ View a painting from the renaissance period of art. Artist to research include Leonardo da Vinci, Michelangelo, Botticelli, Bosch, or El Greco.

Week 2 – Meal Planning

	Breakfast	Lunch	Dinner	Snacks	Goals
Monday					☐ 2 fruit ☐ 1 berry ☐ 5 veggies ☐ 1 cruciferous ☐ 1 leafy green ☐ Legume ☐ Whole grain ☐ Flax/Chia ☐ Nut/Seed
Tuesday					☐ 2 fruit ☐ 1 berry ☐ 5 veggies ☐ 1 cruciferous ☐ 1 leafy green ☐ Legume ☐ Whole grain ☐ Flax/Chia ☐ Nut/Seed
Wednesday					☐ 2 fruit ☐ 1 berry ☐ 5 veggies ☐ 1 cruciferous ☐ 1 leafy green ☐ Legume ☐ Whole grain ☐ Flax/Chia ☐ Nut/Seed
Thursday					☐ 2 fruit ☐ 1 berry ☐ 5 veggies ☐ 1 cruciferous ☐ 1 leafy green ☐ Legume ☐ Whole grain ☐ Flax/Chia ☐ Nut/Seed

	Breakfast	Lunch	Dinner	Snacks	Goals
Friday					☐ 2 fruit ☐ 1 berry ☐ 5 veggies ☐ 1 cruciferous ☐ 1 leafy green ☐ Legume ☐ Whole grain ☐ Flax/Chia ☐ Nut/Seeds
Saturday					☐ 2 fruit ☐ 1 berry ☐ 5 veggies ☐ 1 cruciferous ☐ 1 leafy green ☐ Legume ☐ Whole grain ☐ Flax/Chia ☐ Nut/Seeds
Sunday					☐ 2 fruit ☐ 1 berry ☐ 5 veggies ☐ 1 cruciferous ☐ 1 leafy green ☐ Legume ☐ Whole grain ☐ Flax/Chia ☐ Nut/Seeds

Notes:

_____

_____

_____

Week 2 - Physical Activity

	Sleep	Weights/ Resistance	Steps	Aerobic Exercise	Stretching
Monday					
Tuesday					
Wednesday					
Thursday					
Goals	7-8 Hours	120 min/week (30 min/day three-four times/week)	10,000 steps daily	150 minutes /week	20 minutes /day

	Sleep	Weights/ Resistance	Steps	Aerobic Exercise	Stretching
Friday					
Saturday					
Sunday					
Goals	7-8 Hours	120 min/week (30 min/day three-four times/week)	10,000 steps daily	150 minutes /week	20 minutes /day

Notes

_____

_____

_____

_____

_____

Nature Journal
Week 2

Gratitude Journal

_____

_____

_____

_____

_____

Meditation

☐ Sunday   ☐ Thursday

☐ Monday   ☐ Friday

☐ Tuesday   ☐ Saturday

☐ Wednesday

Additional Notes

_____

_____

_____

_____

_____

_____

_____

_____

_____

Week 3

1) Meal Planning/Log
- ☐ Write recipe name (and cookbook and page number)
- ☐ Check goals against meal plan for the day
- ☐ Create grocery list
- ☐ Make changes to meals if altered so log is accurate

2) Physical Activity
- ☐ Jot hours of sleep night before and any notes
- ☐ Document weight training (if applicable)
- ☐ Document aerobic exercise
- ☐ Complete stretching
- ☐ Record steps at end of day

3) Complete Toxin Avoidance activity
- ☐ See customized wellness plan for recommended activity

4) Complete Emotional Wellness activity
- ☐ Meditate daily
- ☐ Follow emotional wellness plan

5) (Optional) Write Spiritual Letter
- ☐ Complete a spiritual letter theme

6) Nature Journal
- ☐ Commit to 30 mins/day outside. Use the journal to jot your thoughts/drawings for the week.

7) Art/Beauty/Music Appreciation
- ☐ Listen to a piece of classical music. Composers could include Haydn, Mozart, Beethoven or Schubert.

Week 3 – Meal Planning

	Breakfast	Lunch	Dinner	Snacks	Goals
Monday					☐ 2 fruit ☐ 1 berry ☐ 5 veggies ☐ 1 cruciferous ☐ 1 leafy green ☐ Legume ☐ Whole grain ☐ Flax/Chia ☐ Nut/Seed
Tuesday					☐ 2 fruit ☐ 1 berry ☐ 5 veggies ☐ 1 cruciferous ☐ 1 leafy green ☐ Legume ☐ Whole grain ☐ Flax/Chia ☐ Nut/Seed
Wednesday					☐ 2 fruit ☐ 1 berry ☐ 5 veggies ☐ 1 cruciferous ☐ 1 leafy green ☐ Legume ☐ Whole grain ☐ Flax/Chia ☐ Nut/Seed
Thursday					☐ 2 fruit ☐ 1 berry ☐ 5 veggies ☐ 1 cruciferous ☐ 1 leafy green ☐ Legume ☐ Whole grain ☐ Flax/Chia ☐ Nut/Seed

	Breakfast	Lunch	Dinner	Snacks	Goals
Friday					☐ 2 fruit ☐ 1 berry ☐ 5 veggies ☐ 1 cruciferous ☐ 1 leafy green ☐ Legume ☐ Whole grain ☐ Flax/Chia ☐ Nut/Seeds
Saturday					☐ 2 fruit ☐ 1 berry ☐ 5 veggies ☐ 1 cruciferous ☐ 1 leafy green ☐ Legume ☐ Whole grain ☐ Flax/Chia ☐ Nut/Seeds
Sunday					☐ 2 fruit ☐ 1 berry ☐ 5 veggies ☐ 1 cruciferous ☐ 1 leafy green ☐ Legume ☐ Whole grain ☐ Flax/Chia ☐ Nut/Seeds

Notes:

_____

_____

_____

Week 3 - Physical Activity

	Sleep	Weights/ Resistance	Steps	Aerobic Exercise	Stretching
Monday					
Tuesday					
Wednesday					
Thursday					
Goals	7-8 Hours	120 min/week (30 min/day three-four times/week)	10,000 steps daily	150 minutes /week	20 minutes /day

	Sleep	Weights/ Resistance	Steps	Aerobic Exercise	Stretching
Friday					
Saturday					
Sunday					
Goals	7-8 Hours	120 min/week (30 min/day three-four times/week)	10,000 steps daily	150 minutes /week	20 minutes /day

Notes

_____

_____

_____

_____

_____

Nature Journal
Week 3

Gratitude Journal

_____

_____

_____

_____

_____

Meditation

☐ Sunday   ☐ Thursday

☐ Monday   ☐ Friday

☐ Tuesday   ☐ Saturday

☐ Wednesday

Additional Notes

_____

_____

_____

_____

_____

_____

_____

_____

_____

Week 4

1) Meal Planning/Log
- [ ] Write recipe name (and cookbook and page number)
- [ ] Check goals against meal plan for the day
- [ ] Create grocery list
- [ ] Make changes to meals if altered so log is accurate

2) Physical Activity
- [ ] Jot hours of sleep night before and any notes
- [ ] Document weight training (if applicable)
- [ ] Document aerobic exercise
- [ ] Complete stretching
- [ ] Record steps at end of day

3) Complete Toxin Avoidance activity
- [ ] See customized wellness plan for recommended activity

4) Complete Emotional Wellness activity
- [ ] Meditate daily
- [ ] Follow emotional wellness plan

5) (Optional) Write Spiritual Letter
- [ ] Complete a spiritual letter theme

6) Nature Journal
- [ ] Commit to 30 mins/day outside. Use the journal to jot your thoughts/drawings for the week.

7) Art/Beauty/Music Appreciation
- [ ] Focus on the beauty of moving water. Whether this is the image of an ocean tide, or a waterfall, or a stream.

Week 4 – Meal Planning

	Breakfast	Lunch	Dinner	Snacks	Goals
Monday					☐ 2 fruit ☐ 1 berry ☐ 5 veggies ☐ 1 cruciferous ☐ 1 leafy green ☐ Legume ☐ Whole grain ☐ Flax/Chia ☐ Nut/Seed
Tuesday					☐ 2 fruit ☐ 1 berry ☐ 5 veggies ☐ 1 cruciferous ☐ 1 leafy green ☐ Legume ☐ Whole grain ☐ Flax/Chia ☐ Nut/Seed
Wednesday					☐ 2 fruit ☐ 1 berry ☐ 5 veggies ☐ 1 cruciferous ☐ 1 leafy green ☐ Legume ☐ Whole grain ☐ Flax/Chia ☐ Nut/Seed
Thursday					☐ 2 fruit ☐ 1 berry ☐ 5 veggies ☐ 1 cruciferous ☐ 1 leafy green ☐ Legume ☐ Whole grain ☐ Flax/Chia ☐ Nut/Seed

	Breakfast	Lunch	Dinner	Snacks	Goals
Friday					☐ 2 fruit ☐ 1 berry ☐ 5 veggies ☐ 1 cruciferous ☐ 1 leafy green ☐ Legume ☐ Whole grain ☐ Flax/Chia ☐ Nut/Seeds
Saturday					☐ 2 fruit ☐ 1 berry ☐ 5 veggies ☐ 1 cruciferous ☐ 1 leafy green ☐ Legume ☐ Whole grain ☐ Flax/Chia ☐ Nut/Seeds
Sunday					☐ 2 fruit ☐ 1 berry ☐ 5 veggies ☐ 1 cruciferous ☐ 1 leafy green ☐ Legume ☐ Whole grain ☐ Flax/Chia ☐ Nut/Seeds

Notes:

_____

_____

_____

Week 4 - Physical Activity

	Sleep	Weights/ Resistance	Steps	Aerobic Exercise	Stretching
Monday					
Tuesday					
Wednesday					
Thursday					
Goals	7-8 Hours	120 min/week (30 min/day three-four times/week)	10,000 steps daily	150 minutes /week	20 minutes /day

	Sleep	Weights/ Resistance	Steps	Aerobic Exercise	Stretching
Friday					
Saturday					
Sunday					
Goals	7-8 Hours	120 min/week (30 min/day three-four times/week)	10,000 steps daily	150 minutes /week	20 minutes /day

Notes

_____

_____

_____

_____

_____

Nature Journal
Week 4

Gratitude Journal

_____

_____

_____

_____

_____

Meditation

☐ Sunday   ☐ Thursday

☐ Monday   ☐ Friday

☐ Tuesday   ☐ Saturday

☐ Wednesday

Additional Notes

_____

_____

_____

_____

_____

_____

_____

_____

_____

Week 5

1) Meal Planning/Log
- ☐ Write recipe name (and cookbook and page number)
- ☐ Check goals against meal plan for the day
- ☐ Create grocery list
- ☐ Make changes to meals if altered so log is accurate

2) Physical Activity
- ☐ Jot hours of sleep night before and any notes
- ☐ Document weight training (if applicable)
- ☐ Document aerobic exercise
- ☐ Complete stretching
- ☐ Record steps at end of day

3) Complete Toxin Avoidance activity
- ☐ See customized wellness plan for recommended activity

4) Complete Emotional Wellness activity
- ☐ Meditate daily
- ☐ Follow emotional wellness plan

5) (Optional) Write Spiritual Letter
- ☐ Complete a spiritual letter theme

6) Nature Journal
- ☐ Commit to 30 mins/day outside. Use the journal to jot your thoughts/drawings for the week.

7) Art/Beauty/Music Appreciation
- ☐ Listen to a piece of music from the romantic period. Composers include Debussy, Chopin, Liszt, and Verdi.

Week 5 – Meal Planning

	Breakfast	Lunch	Dinner	Snacks	Goals
Monday					☐ 2 fruit ☐ 1 berry ☐ 5 veggies ☐ 1 cruciferous ☐ 1 leafy green ☐ Legume ☐ Whole grain ☐ Flax/Chia ☐ Nut/Seed
Tuesday					☐ 2 fruit ☐ 1 berry ☐ 5 veggies ☐ 1 cruciferous ☐ 1 leafy green ☐ Legume ☐ Whole grain ☐ Flax/Chia ☐ Nut/Seed
Wednesday					☐ 2 fruit ☐ 1 berry ☐ 5 veggies ☐ 1 cruciferous ☐ 1 leafy green ☐ Legume ☐ Whole grain ☐ Flax/Chia ☐ Nut/Seed
Thursday					☐ 2 fruit ☐ 1 berry ☐ 5 veggies ☐ 1 cruciferous ☐ 1 leafy green ☐ Legume ☐ Whole grain ☐ Flax/Chia ☐ Nut/Seed

	Breakfast	Lunch	Dinner	Snacks	Goals
Friday					☐ 2 fruit ☐ 1 berry ☐ 5 veggies ☐ 1 cruciferous ☐ 1 leafy green ☐ Legume ☐ Whole grain ☐ Flax/Chia ☐ Nut/Seeds
Saturday					☐ 2 fruit ☐ 1 berry ☐ 5 veggies ☐ 1 cruciferous ☐ 1 leafy green ☐ Legume ☐ Whole grain ☐ Flax/Chia ☐ Nut/Seeds
Sunday					☐ 2 fruit ☐ 1 berry ☐ 5 veggies ☐ 1 cruciferous ☐ 1 leafy green ☐ Legume ☐ Whole grain ☐ Flax/Chia ☐ Nut/Seeds

Notes:

_____

_____

_____

Week 5 - Physical Activity

	Sleep	Weights/ Resistance	Steps	Aerobic Exercise	Stretching
Monday					
Tuesday					
Wednesday					
Thursday					
Goals	7-8 Hours	120 min/week (30 min/day three-four times/week)	10,000 steps daily	150 minutes /week	20 minutes /day

	Sleep	Weights/ Resistance	Steps	Aerobic Exercise	Stretching
Friday					
Saturday					
Sunday					
Goals	7-8 Hours	120 min/week (30 min/day three-four times/week)	10,000 steps daily	150 minutes /week	20 minutes /day

Notes

_____

_____

_____

_____

_____

Nature Journal
Week 5

Gratitude Journal

_____

_____

_____

_____

_____

Meditation

☐ Sunday   ☐ Thursday

☐ Monday   ☐ Friday

☐ Tuesday   ☐ Saturday

☐ Wednesday

Additional Notes

_____

_____

_____

_____

_____

_____

_____

_____

_____

Week 6

1) Meal Planning/Log
- ☐ Write recipe name (and cookbook and page number)
- ☐ Check goals against meal plan for the day
- ☐ Create grocery list
- ☐ Make changes to meals if altered so log is accurate

2) Physical Activity
- ☐ Jot hours of sleep night before and any notes
- ☐ Document weight training (if applicable)
- ☐ Document aerobic exercise
- ☐ Complete stretching
- ☐ Record steps at end of day

3) Complete Toxin Avoidance activity
- ☐ See customized wellness plan for recommended activity

4) Complete Emotional Wellness activity
- ☐ Meditate daily
- ☐ Follow emotional wellness plan

5) (Optional) Write Spiritual Letter
- ☐ Complete a spiritual letter theme

6) Nature Journal
- ☐ Commit to 30 mins/day outside. Use the journal to jot your thoughts/drawings for the week.

7) Art/Beauty/Music Appreciation
- ☐ Look at a piece of art from the impressionism movement. Artist include Monet, Renoir, Pissarro, Degas, Cezanne or Matisse.

Week 6 – Meal Planning

	Breakfast	Lunch	Dinner	Snacks	Goals
Monday					☐ 2 fruit ☐ 1 berry ☐ 5 veggies ☐ 1 cruciferous ☐ 1 leafy green ☐ Legume ☐ Whole grain ☐ Flax/Chia ☐ Nut/Seed
Tuesday					☐ 2 fruit ☐ 1 berry ☐ 5 veggies ☐ 1 cruciferous ☐ 1 leafy green ☐ Legume ☐ Whole grain ☐ Flax/Chia ☐ Nut/Seed
Wednesday					☐ 2 fruit ☐ 1 berry ☐ 5 veggies ☐ 1 cruciferous ☐ 1 leafy green ☐ Legume ☐ Whole grain ☐ Flax/Chia ☐ Nut/Seed
Thursday					☐ 2 fruit ☐ 1 berry ☐ 5 veggies ☐ 1 cruciferous ☐ 1 leafy green ☐ Legume ☐ Whole grain ☐ Flax/Chia ☐ Nut/Seed

	Breakfast	Lunch	Dinner	Snacks	Goals
Friday					☐ 2 fruit ☐ 1 berry ☐ 5 veggies ☐ 1 cruciferous ☐ 1 leafy green ☐ Legume ☐ Whole grain ☐ Flax/Chia ☐ Nut/Seeds
Saturday					☐ 2 fruit ☐ 1 berry ☐ 5 veggies ☐ 1 cruciferous ☐ 1 leafy green ☐ Legume ☐ Whole grain ☐ Flax/Chia ☐ Nut/Seeds
Sunday					☐ 2 fruit ☐ 1 berry ☐ 5 veggies ☐ 1 cruciferous ☐ 1 leafy green ☐ Legume ☐ Whole grain ☐ Flax/Chia ☐ Nut/Seeds

Notes:

_____

_____

_____

Week 6 - Physical Activity

	Sleep	Weights/ Resistance	Steps	Aerobic Exercise	Stretching
Monday					
Tuesday					
Wednesday					
Thursday					
Goals	7-8 Hours	120 min/week (30 min/day three-four times/week)	10,000 steps daily	150 minutes /week	20 minutes /day

	Sleep	Weights/ Resistance	Steps	Aerobic Exercise	Stretching
Friday					
Saturday					
Sunday					
Goals	7-8 Hours	120 min/week (30 min/day three-four times/week)	10,000 steps daily	150 minutes /week	20 minutes /day

Notes

_____

_____

_____

_____

_____

Nature Journal
Week 6

Gratitude Journal

_____

_____

_____

_____

_____

Meditation

☐ Sunday   ☐ Thursday

☐ Monday   ☐ Friday

☐ Tuesday   ☐ Saturday

☐ Wednesday

Additional Notes

_____

_____

_____

_____

_____

_____

_____

_____

_____

Week 7

1) Meal Planning/Log
- ☐ Write recipe name (and cookbook and page number)
- ☐ Check goals against meal plan for the day
- ☐ Create grocery list
- ☐ Make changes to meals if altered so log is accurate

2) Physical Activity
- ☐ Jot hours of sleep night before and any notes
- ☐ Document weight training (if applicable)
- ☐ Document aerobic exercise
- ☐ Complete stretching
- ☐ Record steps at end of day

3) Complete Toxin Avoidance activity
- ☐ See customized wellness plan for recommended activity

4) Complete Emotional Wellness activity
- ☐ Meditate daily
- ☐ Follow emotional wellness plan

5) (Optional) Write Spiritual Letter
- ☐ Complete a spiritual letter theme

6) Nature Journal
- ☐ Commit to 30 mins/day outside. Use the journal to jot your thoughts/drawings for the week.

7) Art/Beauty/Music Appreciation
- ☐ Look at a beautiful piece of photography. Reflect on why it inspires you.

Week 7 – Meal Planning

	Breakfast	Lunch	Dinner	Snacks	Goals
Monday					☐ 2 fruit ☐ 1 berry ☐ 5 veggies ☐ 1 cruciferous ☐ 1 leafy green ☐ Legume ☐ Whole grain ☐ Flax/Chia ☐ Nut/Seed
Tuesday					☐ 2 fruit ☐ 1 berry ☐ 5 veggies ☐ 1 cruciferous ☐ 1 leafy green ☐ Legume ☐ Whole grain ☐ Flax/Chia ☐ Nut/Seed
Wednesday					☐ 2 fruit ☐ 1 berry ☐ 5 veggies ☐ 1 cruciferous ☐ 1 leafy green ☐ Legume ☐ Whole grain ☐ Flax/Chia ☐ Nut/Seed
Thursday					☐ 2 fruit ☐ 1 berry ☐ 5 veggies ☐ 1 cruciferous ☐ 1 leafy green ☐ Legume ☐ Whole grain ☐ Flax/Chia ☐ Nut/Seed

	Breakfast	Lunch	Dinner	Snacks	Goals
Friday					☐ 2 fruit ☐ 1 berry ☐ 5 veggies ☐ 1 cruciferous ☐ 1 leafy green ☐ Legume ☐ Whole grain ☐ Flax/Chia ☐ Nut/Seeds
Saturday					☐ 2 fruit ☐ 1 berry ☐ 5 veggies ☐ 1 cruciferous ☐ 1 leafy green ☐ Legume ☐ Whole grain ☐ Flax/Chia ☐ Nut/Seeds
Sunday					☐ 2 fruit ☐ 1 berry ☐ 5 veggies ☐ 1 cruciferous ☐ 1 leafy green ☐ Legume ☐ Whole grain ☐ Flax/Chia ☐ Nut/Seeds

Notes:

_____

_____

_____

Week 7 - Physical Activity

	Sleep	Weights/ Resistance	Steps	Aerobic Exercise	Stretching
Monday					
Tuesday					
Wednesday					
Thursday					
Goals	7-8 Hours	120 min/week (30 min/day three-four times/week)	10,000 steps daily	150 minutes /week	20 minutes /day

	Sleep	Weights/ Resistance	Steps	Aerobic Exercise	Stretching
Friday					
Saturday					
Sunday					
Goals	7-8 Hours	120 min/week (30 min/day three-four times/week)	10,000 steps daily	150 minutes /week	20 minutes /day

Notes

_____

_____

_____

_____

_____

Nature Journal
Week 7

Gratitude Journal

_____

_____

_____

_____

_____

Meditation

☐ Sunday   ☐ Thursday

☐ Monday   ☐ Friday

☐ Tuesday   ☐ Saturday

☐ Wednesday

Additional Notes

_____

_____

_____

_____

_____

_____

_____

_____

_____

Week 8

1) Meal Planning/Log
- ☐ Write recipe name (and cookbook and page number)
- ☐ Check goals against meal plan for the day
- ☐ Create grocery list
- ☐ Make changes to meals if altered so log is accurate

2) Physical Activity
- ☐ Jot hours of sleep night before and any notes
- ☐ Document weight training (if applicable)
- ☐ Document aerobic exercise
- ☐ Complete stretching
- ☐ Record steps at end of day

3) Complete Toxin Avoidance activity
- ☐ See customized wellness plan for recommended activity

4) Complete Emotional Wellness activity
- ☐ Meditate daily
- ☐ Follow emotional wellness plan

5) (Optional) Write Spiritual Letter
- ☐ Complete a spiritual letter theme

6) Nature Journal
- ☐ Commit to 30 mins/day outside. Use the journal to jot your thoughts/drawings for the week.

7) Art/Beauty/Music Appreciation
- ☐ Listen to the trees in the wind. Watch the movement of the trees.

Week 8 – Meal Planning

	Breakfast	Lunch	Dinner	Snacks	Goals
Monday					☐ 2 fruit ☐ 1 berry ☐ 5 veggies ☐ 1 cruciferous ☐ 1 leafy green ☐ Legume ☐ Whole grain ☐ Flax/Chia ☐ Nut/Seed
Tuesday					☐ 2 fruit ☐ 1 berry ☐ 5 veggies ☐ 1 cruciferous ☐ 1 leafy green ☐ Legume ☐ Whole grain ☐ Flax/Chia ☐ Nut/Seed
Wednesday					☐ 2 fruit ☐ 1 berry ☐ 5 veggies ☐ 1 cruciferous ☐ 1 leafy green ☐ Legume ☐ Whole grain ☐ Flax/Chia ☐ Nut/Seed
Thursday					☐ 2 fruit ☐ 1 berry ☐ 5 veggies ☐ 1 cruciferous ☐ 1 leafy green ☐ Legume ☐ Whole grain ☐ Flax/Chia ☐ Nut/Seed

	Breakfast	Lunch	Dinner	Snacks	Goals
Friday					☐ 2 fruit ☐ 1 berry ☐ 5 veggies ☐ 1 cruciferous ☐ 1 leafy green ☐ Legume ☐ Whole grain ☐ Flax/Chia ☐ Nut/Seeds
Saturday					☐ 2 fruit ☐ 1 berry ☐ 5 veggies ☐ 1 cruciferous ☐ 1 leafy green ☐ Legume ☐ Whole grain ☐ Flax/Chia ☐ Nut/Seeds
Sunday					☐ 2 fruit ☐ 1 berry ☐ 5 veggies ☐ 1 cruciferous ☐ 1 leafy green ☐ Legume ☐ Whole grain ☐ Flax/Chia ☐ Nut/Seeds

Notes:

_____

_____

_____

Week 8 - Physical Activity

	Sleep	Weights/ Resistance	Steps	Aerobic Exercise	Stretching
Monday					
Tuesday					
Wednesday					
Thursday					
Goals	7-8 Hours	120 min/week (30 min/day three-four times/week)	10,000 steps daily	150 minutes /week	20 minutes /day

	Sleep	Weights/ Resistance	Steps	Aerobic Exercise	Stretching
Friday					
Saturday					
Sunday					
Goals	7-8 Hours	120 min/week (30 min/day three-four times/week)	10,000 steps daily	150 minutes /week	20 minutes /day

Notes

_____

_____

_____

_____

_____

Nature Journal
Week 8

Gratitude Journal

_____

_____

_____

_____

_____

Meditation

☐ Sunday   ☐ Thursday

☐ Monday   ☐ Friday

☐ Tuesday   ☐ Saturday

☐ Wednesday

Additional Notes

_____

_____

_____

_____

_____

_____

_____

_____

_____

Week 9

1) Meal Planning/Log
- ☐ Write recipe name (and cookbook and page number)
- ☐ Check goals against meal plan for the day
- ☐ Create grocery list
- ☐ Make changes to meals if altered so log is accurate

2) Physical Activity
- ☐ Jot hours of sleep night before and any notes
- ☐ Document weight training (if applicable)
- ☐ Document aerobic exercise
- ☐ Complete stretching
- ☐ Record steps at end of day

3) Complete Toxin Avoidance activity
- ☐ See customized wellness plan for recommended activity

4) Complete Emotional Wellness activity
- ☐ Meditate daily
- ☐ Follow emotional wellness plan

5) (Optional) Write Spiritual Letter
- ☐ Complete a spiritual letter theme

6) Nature Journal
- ☐ Commit to 30 mins/day outside. Use the journal to jot your thoughts/drawings for the week.

7) Art/Beauty/Music Appreciation
- ☐ Listen to one of your favorite pieces of music. Why do you like it? Why is it beautiful to you?

Week 9 – Meal Planning

	Breakfast	Lunch	Dinner	Snacks	Goals
Monday					☐ 2 fruit ☐ 1 berry ☐ 5 veggies ☐ 1 cruciferous ☐ 1 leafy green ☐ Legume ☐ Whole grain ☐ Flax/Chia ☐ Nut/Seed
Tuesday					☐ 2 fruit ☐ 1 berry ☐ 5 veggies ☐ 1 cruciferous ☐ 1 leafy green ☐ Legume ☐ Whole grain ☐ Flax/Chia ☐ Nut/Seed
Wednesday					☐ 2 fruit ☐ 1 berry ☐ 5 veggies ☐ 1 cruciferous ☐ 1 leafy green ☐ Legume ☐ Whole grain ☐ Flax/Chia ☐ Nut/Seed
Thursday					☐ 2 fruit ☐ 1 berry ☐ 5 veggies ☐ 1 cruciferous ☐ 1 leafy green ☐ Legume ☐ Whole grain ☐ Flax/Chia ☐ Nut/Seed

	Breakfast	Lunch	Dinner	Snacks	Goals
Friday					☐ 2 fruit ☐ 1 berry ☐ 5 veggies ☐ 1 cruciferous ☐ 1 leafy green ☐ Legume ☐ Whole grain ☐ Flax/Chia ☐ Nut/Seeds
Saturday					☐ 2 fruit ☐ 1 berry ☐ 5 veggies ☐ 1 cruciferous ☐ 1 leafy green ☐ Legume ☐ Whole grain ☐ Flax/Chia ☐ Nut/Seeds
Sunday					☐ 2 fruit ☐ 1 berry ☐ 5 veggies ☐ 1 cruciferous ☐ 1 leafy green ☐ Legume ☐ Whole grain ☐ Flax/Chia ☐ Nut/Seeds

Notes:

_____

_____

_____

Week 9 - Physical Activity

	Sleep	Weights/ Resistance	Steps	Aerobic Exercise	Stretching
Monday					
Tuesday					
Wednesday					
Thursday					
Goals	7-8 Hours	120 min/week (30 min/day three-four times/week)	10,000 steps daily	150 minutes /week	20 minutes /day

	Sleep	Weights/Resistance	Steps	Aerobic Exercise	Stretching
Friday					
Saturday					
Sunday					
Goals	7-8 Hours	120 min/week (30 min/day three-four times/week)	10,000 steps daily	150 minutes /week	20 minutes /day

Notes

_____

_____

_____

_____

_____

Nature Journal

Week 9

Gratitude Journal

_____

_____

_____

_____

Meditation

☐ Sunday   ☐ Thursday

☐ Monday   ☐ Friday

☐ Tuesday   ☐ Saturday

☐ Wednesday

Additional Notes

_____

_____

_____

_____

_____

_____

_____

_____

Week 10

1) Meal Planning/Log
- ☐ Write recipe name (and cookbook and page number)
- ☐ Check goals against meal plan for the day
- ☐ Create grocery list
- ☐ Make changes to meals if altered so log is accurate

2) Physical Activity
- ☐ Jot hours of sleep night before and any notes
- ☐ Document weight training (if applicable)
- ☐ Document aerobic exercise
- ☐ Complete stretching
- ☐ Record steps at end of day

3) Complete Toxin Avoidance activity
- ☐ See customized wellness plan for recommended activity

4) Complete Emotional Wellness activity
- ☐ Meditate daily
- ☐ Follow emotional wellness plan

5) (Optional) Write Spiritual Letter
- ☐ Complete a spiritual letter theme

6) Nature Journal
- ☐ Commit to 30 mins/day outside. Use the journal to jot your thoughts/drawings for the week.

7) Art/Beauty/Music Appreciation
- ☐ View a sunset this week.

Week 10 – Meal Planning

	Breakfast	Lunch	Dinner	Snacks	Goals
Monday					☐ 2 fruit ☐ 1 berry ☐ 5 veggies ☐ 1 cruciferous ☐ 1 leafy green ☐ Legume ☐ Whole grain ☐ Flax/Chia ☐ Nut/Seed
Tuesday					☐ 2 fruit ☐ 1 berry ☐ 5 veggies ☐ 1 cruciferous ☐ 1 leafy green ☐ Legume ☐ Whole grain ☐ Flax/Chia ☐ Nut/Seed
Wednesday					☐ 2 fruit ☐ 1 berry ☐ 5 veggies ☐ 1 cruciferous ☐ 1 leafy green ☐ Legume ☐ Whole grain ☐ Flax/Chia ☐ Nut/Seed
Thursday					☐ 2 fruit ☐ 1 berry ☐ 5 veggies ☐ 1 cruciferous ☐ 1 leafy green ☐ Legume ☐ Whole grain ☐ Flax/Chia ☐ Nut/Seed

	Breakfast	Lunch	Dinner	Snacks	Goals
Friday					☐ 2 fruit ☐ 1 berry ☐ 5 veggies ☐ 1 cruciferous ☐ 1 leafy green ☐ Legume ☐ Whole grain ☐ Flax/Chia ☐ Nut/Seeds
Saturday					☐ 2 fruit ☐ 1 berry ☐ 5 veggies ☐ 1 cruciferous ☐ 1 leafy green ☐ Legume ☐ Whole grain ☐ Flax/Chia ☐ Nut/Seeds
Sunday					☐ 2 fruit ☐ 1 berry ☐ 5 veggies ☐ 1 cruciferous ☐ 1 leafy green ☐ Legume ☐ Whole grain ☐ Flax/Chia ☐ Nut/Seeds

Notes:

_____

_____

_____

Week 10 - Physical Activity

	Sleep	Weights/ Resistance	Steps	Aerobic Exercise	Stretching
Monday					
Tuesday					
Wednesday					
Thursday					
Goals	7-8 Hours	120 min/week (30 min/day three-four times/week)	10,000 steps daily	150 minutes /week	20 minutes /day

	Sleep	Weights/Resistance	Steps	Aerobic Exercise	Stretching
Friday					
Saturday					
Sunday					
Goals	7-8 Hours	120 min/week (30 min/day three-four times/week)	10,000 steps daily	150 minutes /week	20 minutes /day

Notes

_____

_____

_____

_____

_____

Nature Journal
Week 10

Gratitude Journal

_____

_____

_____

_____

_____

Meditation

☐ Sunday   ☐ Thursday

☐ Monday   ☐ Friday

☐ Tuesday   ☐ Saturday

☐ Wednesday

Additional Notes

_____

_____

_____

_____

_____

_____

_____

_____

_____

Week 11

1) Meal Planning/Log
- [ ] Write recipe name (and cookbook and page number)
- [ ] Check goals against meal plan for the day
- [ ] Create grocery list
- [ ] Make changes to meals if altered so log is accurate

2) Physical Activity
- [ ] Jot hours of sleep night before and any notes
- [ ] Document weight training (if applicable)
- [ ] Document aerobic exercise
- [ ] Complete stretching
- [ ] Record steps at end of day

3) Complete Toxin Avoidance activity
- [ ] See customized wellness plan for recommended activity

4) Complete Emotional Wellness activity
- [ ] Meditate daily
- [ ] Follow emotional wellness plan

5) (Optional) Write Spiritual Letter
- [ ] Complete a spiritual letter theme

6) Nature Journal
- [ ] Commit to 30 mins/day outside. Use the journal to jot your thoughts/drawings for the week.

7) Art/Beauty/Music Appreciation
- [ ] View a sunrise this week.

Week 11 – Meal Planning

	Breakfast	Lunch	Dinner	Snacks	Goals
Monday					☐ 2 fruit ☐ 1 berry ☐ 5 veggies ☐ 1 cruciferous ☐ 1 leafy green ☐ Legume ☐ Whole grain ☐ Flax/Chia ☐ Nut/Seed
Tuesday					☐ 2 fruit ☐ 1 berry ☐ 5 veggies ☐ 1 cruciferous ☐ 1 leafy green ☐ Legume ☐ Whole grain ☐ Flax/Chia ☐ Nut/Seed
Wednesday					☐ 2 fruit ☐ 1 berry ☐ 5 veggies ☐ 1 cruciferous ☐ 1 leafy green ☐ Legume ☐ Whole grain ☐ Flax/Chia ☐ Nut/Seed
Thursday					☐ 2 fruit ☐ 1 berry ☐ 5 veggies ☐ 1 cruciferous ☐ 1 leafy green ☐ Legume ☐ Whole grain ☐ Flax/Chia ☐ Nut/Seed

	Breakfast	Lunch	Dinner	Snacks	Goals
Friday					☐ 2 fruit ☐ 1 berry ☐ 5 veggies ☐ 1 cruciferous ☐ 1 leafy green ☐ Legume ☐ Whole grain ☐ Flax/Chia ☐ Nut/Seeds
Saturday					☐ 2 fruit ☐ 1 berry ☐ 5 veggies ☐ 1 cruciferous ☐ 1 leafy green ☐ Legume ☐ Whole grain ☐ Flax/Chia ☐ Nut/Seeds
Sunday					☐ 2 fruit ☐ 1 berry ☐ 5 veggies ☐ 1 cruciferous ☐ 1 leafy green ☐ Legume ☐ Whole grain ☐ Flax/Chia ☐ Nut/Seeds

Notes:

_____

_____

_____

Week 11 - Physical Activity

	Sleep	Weights/ Resistance	Steps	Aerobic Exercise	Stretching
Monday					
Tuesday					
Wednesday					
Thursday					
Goals	7-8 Hours	120 min/week (30 min/day three-four times/week)	10,000 steps daily	150 minutes /week	20 minutes /day

	Sleep	Weights/ Resistance	Steps	Aerobic Exercise	Stretching
Friday					
Saturday					
Sunday					
Goals	7-8 Hours	120 min/week (30 min/day three-four times/week)	10,000 steps daily	150 minutes /week	20 minutes /day

Notes

_____

_____

_____

_____

_____

Nature Journal
Week 11

Gratitude Journal

_____

_____

_____

_____

_____

Meditation

☐ Sunday   ☐ Thursday

☐ Monday   ☐ Friday

☐ Tuesday   ☐ Saturday

☐ Wednesday

Additional Notes

_____

_____

_____

_____

_____

_____

_____

_____

_____

Week 12

1) Meal Planning/Log
- ☐ Write recipe name (and cookbook and page number)
- ☐ Check goals against meal plan for the day
- ☐ Create grocery list
- ☐ Make changes to meals if altered so log is accurate

2) Physical Activity
- ☐ Jot hours of sleep night before and any notes
- ☐ Document weight training (if applicable)
- ☐ Document aerobic exercise
- ☐ Complete stretching
- ☐ Record steps at end of day

3) Complete Toxin Avoidance activity
- ☐ See customized wellness plan for recommended activity

4) Complete Emotional Wellness activity
- ☐ Meditate daily
- ☐ Follow emotional wellness plan

5) (Optional) Write Spiritual Letter
- ☐ Complete a spiritual letter theme

6) Nature Journal
- ☐ Commit to 30 mins/day outside. Use the journal to jot your thoughts/drawings for the week.

7) Art/Beauty/Music Appreciation
- ☐ Choose an everyday mundane thing and find beauty in it.

Week 12 – Meal Planning

	Breakfast	Lunch	Dinner	Snacks	Goals
Monday					☐ 2 fruit ☐ 1 berry ☐ 5 veggies ☐ 1 cruciferous ☐ 1 leafy green ☐ Legume ☐ Whole grain ☐ Flax/Chia ☐ Nut/Seed
Tuesday					☐ 2 fruit ☐ 1 berry ☐ 5 veggies ☐ 1 cruciferous ☐ 1 leafy green ☐ Legume ☐ Whole grain ☐ Flax/Chia ☐ Nut/Seed
Wednesday					☐ 2 fruit ☐ 1 berry ☐ 5 veggies ☐ 1 cruciferous ☐ 1 leafy green ☐ Legume ☐ Whole grain ☐ Flax/Chia ☐ Nut/Seed
Thursday					☐ 2 fruit ☐ 1 berry ☐ 5 veggies ☐ 1 cruciferous ☐ 1 leafy green ☐ Legume ☐ Whole grain ☐ Flax/Chia ☐ Nut/Seed

	Breakfast	Lunch	Dinner	Snacks	Goals
Friday					☐ 2 fruit ☐ 1 berry ☐ 5 veggies ☐ 1 cruciferous ☐ 1 leafy green ☐ Legume ☐ Whole grain ☐ Flax/Chia ☐ Nut/Seeds
Saturday					☐ 2 fruit ☐ 1 berry ☐ 5 veggies ☐ 1 cruciferous ☐ 1 leafy green ☐ Legume ☐ Whole grain ☐ Flax/Chia ☐ Nut/Seeds
Sunday					☐ 2 fruit ☐ 1 berry ☐ 5 veggies ☐ 1 cruciferous ☐ 1 leafy green ☐ Legume ☐ Whole grain ☐ Flax/Chia ☐ Nut/Seeds

Notes:

_____

_____

_____

Week 12 - Physical Activity

	Sleep	Weights/ Resistance	Steps	Aerobic Exercise	Stretching
Monday					
Tuesday					
Wednesday					
Thursday					
Goals	7-8 Hours	120 min/week (30 min/day three-four times/week)	10,000 steps daily	150 minutes /week	20 minutes /day

	Sleep	Weights/ Resistance	Steps	Aerobic Exercise	Stretching
Friday					
Saturday					
Sunday					
Goals	7-8 Hours	120 min/week (30 min/day three-four times/week)	10,000 steps daily	150 minutes /week	20 minutes /day

Notes

_____

_____

_____

_____

_____

Nature Journal
Week 12

Gratitude Journal

_____

_____

_____

_____

_____

Meditation

☐ Sunday   ☐ Thursday

☐ Monday   ☐ Friday

☐ Tuesday   ☐ Saturday

☐ Wednesday

Additional Notes

_____

_____

_____

_____

_____

_____

_____

_____

Toxin Avoidance

Tobacco Cessation Worksheet

What is this?

This worksheet is intended for all tobacco users with low use. Smokers who did so regularly weekly, daily or multiple times daily response NEED professional assistance. This worksheet may still be helpful, but when you smoke regularly you develop a chemical dependence.

Why do we care?

Smoking causes heart attacks!

Tobacco use is associated with heart disease. "Smoking and tobacco use of any kind increases the risk of developing heart disease. Chemicals in tobacco can cause damage to your heart and blood vessel, leading up to narrowing of the arteries due to plaque build-up (atherosclerosis). Carbon monoxide build up increases heart workload."

"No amount of smoking is safe. It is a dose relationship, meaning the more you smoke the higher the risk. Heart disease risk reduces one year after quitting. Drops almost to that of non-smoker at 15 years of not smoking."[1]

Smoking causes lung cancer!

"Lung cancer is diagnosed 220,000 times each year in the United States. Causes more deaths annually than the next three cancers combined including those of the colon, breast and pancreas. At any given moment, nearly 400,000 Americans are living under lung cancers dark shadow."

Per the American lung Association, smoking tobacco contributes to up to 90% of all lung cancer deaths. "Men who smoke are 23 times more likely and women are 13 times more likely to develop lung cancer than nonsmokers. Non-smokers have a 20 to 30% higher risk of developing lung cancer of the regularly exposed to cigarette smoke."

Smoking causes other chronic disease!

Smoking causes lung disease, meaning asthma, COPD, chronic bronchitis, and emphysema. If you have ever been around someone who has these illnesses, they are some of the worst. They are very debilitating. They make it difficult to hike, climb, walk, even cook and walk around the home. Not these diseases are preventable, but smoking is and is highly associated with lung diseases.

Smoking is also associated with stroke, Alzheimer's dementia.

Smoking is even associated with diabetes. "Smokers are roughly 50% more likely to develop DM than nonsmokers. Heavy smokers are at higher risk."

How often is too much?

Any smoking is too much. When is starting a forest fire too much? Forest fires are hard to control, hard to predict. There are some very skilled firefighters who can mitigate forest fire risk of spread, but an average person doesn't know how to reduce the risk of spread. Smoking is one of the most addictive habits a human being can partake in. In my experience in the ER, many of my patients who have also used crack, cocaine, methamphetamine, and even heroin have said that quitting smoking is one of the hardest things to do.

How much is too much? Why would you ever take the risk that the habit of smoking could turn into a forest fire and become uncontrollable? When you are playing with a habit that's so addictive, hard to quit, and so bad for you, any smoking is too much. If you are smoking rarely, then it should be easy to quite completely. If you are smoking a lot, you will likely undergo some withdrawals and may need professional help.

How to quit?

The American Lung Association has numerous resources to quit smoking. They answer tough questions like what to expect, the challenges you should prepare for and answers to common questions about quitting smoking. Check out their website at https://www.lung.org/stop-smoking/i-want-to-quit/.

Why should I quit?

Start with the following questions and jot down a few responses:

1. What do you enjoy about smoking?

    _____

    _____

    _____

    _____

2. How does smoking impact my life? Health? Financial?

    Convenience? Friends and Family?

    _____

    _____

    _____

    _____

3.	Are there things you could do to replace your urge to smoke with

	something healthier?

	_____

	_____

	_____

	_____

4.	In what ways, would your life be better without smoking?

	_____

	_____

	_____

	_____

Second-Hand Smoke Reduction Worksheet

What is this?

For persons that answered that they were exposed to second-hand smoke monthly, weekly, daily or multiple times daily, we recommend you spend some time with this worksheet.

Second-hand smoke is absolutely associated with increased risks of multiple diseases, but is a sensitive topic. Often, people exposed to second-hand smoke don't have a choice. Furthermore, the people who smoke in our homes and in our lives, are likely people we love and care about. This makes it difficult to be too critical, particularly when we know that this person is already trying hard. Reminding them of the health problems that second-hand smoke creates might help them on their path to quitting.

In addition, I have seen numerous cases in the community of people smoking publicly met with problems on both sides. Sometimes those people are not cautious at all, exposing everyone around them to the smoke. In other cases, I've seen people trying to avoid the smoke yelling at smokers, who might be addicted to the habit, have chemical dependence or who are trying to be discrete but can't be due to circumstance. We all need to be sensitive to these circumstances. Try and pause and think of life through the lens of the people we share our communities with. Try and avoid harsh judgment and recognize that a small amount of second-hand smoke exposure is unlikely to cause significant harm.

Another large area of highly under-appreciated second-hand smoke exposure comes from cooking, particularly with animal products, animal fats and oils.

Why do we care?

Frying meat causes cancer!

Regular cooking of fried products is associated with cancer.

"Cancer risk depends on what's being fried. A study of women in China found that smokers who stir fried meat every day had nearly 3 times the odds of lung cancer compared to smokers who stir fried foods other than meat on a daily basis."

Cutting down on cooking any fried items certainly would reduce your risk of cancer. In addition, as you have already learned in nutrition, eating a plant-based diet has numerous health benefits. One benefit is that you shouldn't ever be frying meat. This will cut down on your exposure as well.

Inhaling Someone Else's Tobacco Smoke Causes Lung Cancer!
The U.S. Environmental Protection Agency, the U.S. National Toxicology Program, the U.S. Surgeon General, and the International Agency for Research on Cancer have all classified secondhand smoke as a known human carcinogen (a cancer-causing agent).

The Surgeon General estimates that, during 2005-2009, secondhand smoke exposure caused more than 7,300 lung cancer deaths among adult nonsmokers each year.

Exposure to second-hand smoke continues to decline in public places, thanks to policies enacted by the Federal and State Governments to reduce exposure. This has had a dramatic impact on all of our risk of inhaling someone else's tobacco smoke.

Inhaling Someone Else's Tobacco Smoke Causes Other Cancers!

Some research also suggests that secondhand smoke may increase the risk of breast cancer, nasal sinus cavity cancer, and <u>nasopharyngeal cancer</u> in adults[3] and the risk of <u>leukemia</u>, <u>lymphoma</u>, and brain tumors in children.

How much is too much?

This is a very challenging issue for a lot of people. Any smoke inhalation is potentially harmful. Obviously, there is a dose-response relationship, meaning that the more you are exposed to second-hand smoke, the worse things become for you. However, we have to keep in mind that smoking is one of the strongest addictions we have as humans. Those that smoke around us may be chemically and psychologically dependent on smoking.

Pointing out the facts as above can help curb smoking or even prompt people to quit. Love and tolerance is required in approaching this sensitive topic.

What can I do?

Start with the following questions and jot down a few responses:

1. Where am I exposed to second-hand smoke?

    _____

    _____

    _____

    _____

2. Who exposes me to second-hand smoke?

    _____

    _____

_____

_____

3. Are there ways to avoid exposure to second-hand smoke?

_____

_____

_____

_____

4. Are there opportunities to encourage and support someone else in their effort to stop smoking?

_____

_____

_____

_____

Alcohol Use Worksheet

What is this?

For persons that answered that they use alcohol monthly, weekly, daily or multiple times daily, we recommend you spend some time with this worksheet.

Binge drinking is defined as drinking more than 3 drinks in one sitting.

At risk drinking is > 2 for a man and > 1 for a female. This means that if at any given point you are consuming > 1 for a female or > 2 for a man, you are at risk of development of an alcohol use problem.

Why do we care?

Alcohol is associated with numerous chronic diseases, not to mention it can prevent you from achieving your maximal potential. There has been literature that supports the use of very moderate alcohol consumption 1-2 for male and 1 for female, but no more than that. Many Americans will not consume any alcohol on some days and then 3-4 or more on the weekends or pleasure days. This is binge drinking. It is associated with liver disease, kidney disease, heart attacks, stroke, high blood pressure and high cholesterol. It is also associated with cancers and pancreatitis.

A huge part of alcohol use relates to mental health. When we have poor mental health, we often use too much alcohol. This can result in the "self-treating" phenomenon where we use alcohol to curb anxiety, take the edge off, relax, or even treat the blues. This is a recipe for disaster, as the dose required for this effect increases rapidly, even in days. In addition, the withdrawal is worse than the benefit. Meaning when you stop drinking, things get worse.

We should never drink for an alcohol effect, as this effect will continue to elude us, resulting in alcohol dependence.

How much is too much?

Alcohol is highly addictive with potentially life-threatening withdrawal. Most people who drink more than 1 for a woman and 2 for a man will experience mild withdrawal symptoms. Those symptoms can be as minor as irritability or sleep disturbance.

They can be major such as alcohol withdrawal tachycardia, high blood pressure emergency, stroke, seizures. The guidelines above should protect you from development of stomach, liver, cardiac disease. You can develop liver disease, enlarged heart, arrhythmias, kidney disease, stomach disease and numerous cancers from too much consumption.

What can I do?

Start with the following questions and jot down a few responses:

1. How often do I drink alcohol?

_____

_____

_____

_____

2. Why do I drink alcohol?

_____

_____

3. Do I ever drink more than 2 for a male and 1 for a female? When do I do this?

_____

_____

_____

_____

4. What can I do to make sure that I never consume more than 1 for female and 2 for male? Are there days I can avoid drinking altogether?

_____

_____

_____

_____

Filtered Water Worksheet

What is this?

Drinking filtered water is good for your health, if it's not out of a plastic bottle.

You have likely been referred to this worksheet, if you answered that you are not currently drinking filtered water.

Why do we care?

In 2009, the EPA warned that "threats to drinking water are increasing."[1]

Everyone has heard about the lead contamination in Flint, Michigan. There are risks from other heavy metals. In 2010, EWG released a landmark report warning that chromium-6, a human carcinogen (cancer-causing), was found in the drinking water of 200 million Americans.[1] Harvard University found unsafe levels of polyfluoroakyl and PFASs (perfluoroalkyl substances), both known to cause cancer and disrupt hormones in the drinking water of 6 million Americans.[1]

Finally, there are biologic diseases transmitted via contaminated water sources. If you live in a rural area with a well, you should have your well tested. If there is a biologic threat, it could be from neighboring farms, often who maintain too many head of livestock per space area. One of the more notable biologic outbreaks into water happened in 1993 in Milwaukee, Wisconsin. I remember this outbreak, as I grew up there. Cryptosporidium got into the water sources and sickened 400,000 people and killed 100.[1]

---

[1] https://www.mnn.com/earth-matters/translating-uncle-sam/stories/how-polluted-is-us-drinking-water. Accessed May 21st, 2019.

What can be done?

Buying water bottles is never a good idea. Plastic, as we will learn, is very bad for the environment and often contains hormone disrupting chemicals. In fact, one could argue that you are better drinking unfiltered water than plastic bottle water.

The best option is to filter your own water in your home. There are several ways to do this at multiple different costs. Perhaps, the easiest and least annoying way to do it is to have a reverse osmosis system installed at your home sink off from your water line. It comes with a separate faucet, which is where you dispense your filtered water. In addition, this water line, now filtered, should be connected to your ice machine.

This can be costly, but it varies. Home Depot and Lowe's offer systems in the $200-$300 range, which for a handy person can be very easy to install. I've done them myself. They do have to have regular filter change outs, which can be costly. Sometimes as frequently as every 6-12 months.

Another, less expensive approach is a filter that goes on the faucet. It can be turned on or off, depending on what you are doing. If you are washing fruits/vegetables, the water should be filtered. If you are boiling hot water, you don't necessarily need to filter it. One could argue that even washing your hands should be done with the safest, filtered water. If you are pre-washing dishes or watering the plants, then unfiltered may be a better choice.

Finally, you can purchase a Brita or similar brand filter for drinking water. You essentially pour the water in the top and gravity does the rest. Over the course of several minutes the water drops through the filter on the pitcher into a lower chamber, now available for drinking.

What can I do?

Start with the following questions and jot down a few responses:

1. How often do I drink non-filtered water?

_____

_____

_____

_____

2. Why do I drink unfiltered water?

_____

_____

_____

_____

3. Are there times that I drink filtered water? Brita like filtered pitcher? Reverse Osmosis? Central Home Filtration?

_____

_____

_____

_____

_____

4. What can I do to increase the consumption of filtered water for myself? For my family?

_____

_____

_____

_____

_____

Plastics Worksheet

What is this?

You answered that you may not always use BPA free plastics.

Plastics are a relatively newer part of our life. Our ancestors used ceramic, metal, and even gourds to keep food products, water, etc. When we consider the uses for plastics, they have been very convenient, saving use time.

They are not typically good for the environment though. In addition, they are coming into close contact with our bodies, sometimes in the wearable form, but often as it relates to storage of drinking water and food. BPAs or bisphenyl A's have been found in plastics and are associated with hormone disruption, particularly bad for men, causing feminization, but also bad for women exposing them to risk of hormonal cancers, like some breast cancers.

Why do we care?

BPA has been in plastics since the 1960s.[2] It has been found in plastics, such as water bottles, but also in can liners for canned goods, and even dental composites.[1]

BPAs have been linked to possible health effects on the brain, behavior, prostate gland of fetuses, infants, and children.[1] There may even be a link to blood pressure.[1]

What can be done?

---

[2] "What is BPA, and what are the concerns about BPA?" Brent Bauer, MD. "Healthy Lifestyle. Mayo Clinic. https://www.mayoclinic.org/healthy-lifestyle/nutrition-and-healthy-eating/expert-answers/bpa/faq-20058331. Accessed May 21st, 2019.

We should try and use BPA-free products whenever we can. Specifically, when you buy any plastic products, look for BPA-free logo or indicator. If it doesn't have it, don't buy it.

Dispose all your unlabeled or unknown plastics in the home. It's a shame, but if you aren't sure, it's got to go.

In addition, be careful when buying canned goods. Canned foods are the only reasonable option for some to get the beans, legumes, fruits and vegetables. Personally, I prefer fresh and with the advent of the InstaPot™ and beans ready within a couple of hours, it's far better to stored dried beans and avoid canned goods altogether. If you do need to consume canned goods though, check for BPA-free labeling.

If possible, try and avoid plastics altogether, if there is a reasonable alternative to what you are purchasing.

When cooking with plastics, be sure to avoid any heat. If you must microwave a dish, use ceramic or glass, never microwave with plastic.

What can I do?

Start with the following questions and jot down a few responses:

1. How often do I use plastic? How often am I aware of the BPA status of plastic?

   _____

   _____

   _____

   _____

2. Why do I use plastic? Why do I use unknown BPA status plastic?

_____

_____

_____

_____

3. Are there times where I use alternatives to plastic? Are there things that I can do to clean up the home, reducing plastic exposures?

_____

_____

_____

_____

_____

4. What can I do to reduce exposure to canned goods? Plastics? When I do buy plastic goods, how can I remember to make sure it's BPA free?

_____

_____

_____

_____

_____

Smog, Air Quality, or Pollution Exposure Reduction Worksheet

What is this?

This worksheet is intended for all persons that answered that they are exposed to **Smog, Air Quality, or Pollution Exposure Reduction Worksheet** 60-90 minutes, 90-120 minutes, or > 120 minutes of daily exposure.

According to the American Heart Association, "Pollution can come from traffic, factories, power generation, wildfires, or even cooking with a wood stove."

Why do we care?

Air Pollution Causes Heart Attacks!

"Someone with atherosclerosis (vessel plaques) ...experiences immediate trouble when pollutants play a role in causing plaque in a blood vessel to rupture, triggering a heart attack."[1]

Air Pollution Causes Inflammation!

"Pollution is also believed to have inflammatory effects on the heart, causing chronic cardiovascular problems."[1]

Air Pollution Causes Lung Disease!

Emphysema and chronic bronchitis are two forms of lung disease. "Chronic Lung Disease affects more than 24 million Americans according to the CDC. Smoking is the leading cause but also air pollution may play a role."

Air Pollution May Cause Other Diseases!

"The risk of death is greater from long-term exposure. Current science suggests air pollution facilitates atherosclerosis development and progression, said the scientific panel that worked on the statement. It also may play a role in high blood pressure, heart failure, and diabetes."[1]

Check out this YouTube Video to learn more about the impact of air pollution: https://youtu.be/9jOpNF2uc2M.

How often is too much?

We need to be careful never to fear going outside, because fresh air, time in nature are all important to health and well-being. Wellness must include time outdoors. For some of us, we live in a city and time outdoors, means time in smog or air pollution. We can't control where we live, some of the time, and we can't control when we have to go to work or be outside sometimes.

We can, however, control when we go outside for pleasure. We should watch smog ratings and air quality indices for warnings regarding air pollution. When they show potential problems, we need to avoid going outdoors.

How to avoid it?

It's impossible to avoid air quality problems completely. Using tools can be helpful.

Air Now is a helpful tool to assessing your communities air quality. https://airnow.gov.

Consider planning your day's outdoor activities for fun or leisure, by checking with this helpful website. If you are able to travel somewhere in a brief time to enjoy outdoor activities that would be best.

How can I curb my behaviors to reduce risk of pollution exposure?

Start with the following questions and jot down a few responses:

1. Where are you exposed to smog, air pollution, or air quality problems?

   _____

   _____

   _____

   _____

2. What can you do to reduce the exposures you listed above?

   _____

   _____

   _____

   _____

3. Could you travel to an area with cleaner air to enjoy outdoor activities?

   _____

   _____

_____

_____

4. What ways can you advocate for clean air in your communities?

_____

_____

_____

_____

Indoor Pollution Exposure Reduction Worksheet

What is this?

This worksheet is intended for all persons that answered that they are exposed to **Indoor wood smoke, cooking smoke, or other indoor quality problems** 60-90 minutes, 90-120 minutes, or > 120 minutes of daily exposure.

According to the American Heart Association, "Pollution can come from traffic, factories, power generation, wildfires, or even cooking with a wood stove."

Most of us are exposed to air pollution of some sort, but air pollution in the home is particularly difficult to avoid.

Why do we care?

Air Pollution from Cooking Meat Causes Cancer!

Frying foods is a health risk with most cooking oils, although some oils are better than others. Check out Dr. Michael Greger's video on frying foods. https://youtu.be/i6vdycYq3SI . Cancer risk depends on what's being fried. A study of women in China found that smokers who stir fried meat every day had nearly 3 times the odds of lung cancer compared to smokers who stir fried foods other than meat on a daily basis.

Air Pollution Causes Heart Attacks!

"Someone with atherosclerosis (vessel plaques) ...experiences immediate trouble when pollutants play a role in causing plaque in a blood vessel to rupture, triggering a heart attack."[1]

Air Pollution Causes Inflammation!

"Pollution is also believed to have inflammatory effects on the heart, causing chronic cardiovascular problems."[1]

Air Pollution Causes Lung Disease!

Emphysema and chronic bronchitis are two forms of lung disease. "Chronic Lung Disease affects more than 24 million Americans according to the CDC. Smoking is the leading cause but also air pollution may play a role."

Air Pollution May Cause Other Diseases!

"The risk of death is greater from long-term exposure. Current science suggests air pollution facilitates atherosclerosis development and progression, said the scientific panel that worked on the statement. It also may play a role in high blood pressure, heart failure, and diabetes."[1]

Check out this YouTube Video to learn more about the impact of air pollution: https://youtu.be/9jOpNF2uc2M.

How often is too much?

When we go outside, we can use tools to help us determine the amount of air pollution in the air, but that's not easy for indoor air pollution.

It's very difficult to control what we are exposed to inside of the home. I think it's more helpful to look at several different air quality issues in the home.

How to avoid it?

It's impossible to avoid air quality problems completely. Using tools can be helpful. Here are a few ideas regarding indoor air quality.

- Do you use wood stove/pellet stove/coal stove in the home? If so, are they near your bedrooms? If you can get rid of these exposures and substitute for healthier ways to heat the home, then do so. If you can't, then consider sleeping in a separate room, away from the heating element. In addition, consider buying an air purifier to cleanse the air. We like the Germ Guardian unit: https://amzn.to/2VlcLtz. Check it out. You do need to change the filters regularly.
- Do you cook with oil? Be sure to check out the above video and learn about safer oils to cook with. If you can reduce cooking with oil, please do so. Try never to fry animal products, like eggs, meat, etc. If you do have to fry vegetables and other foods, then consider a strong fume/smoke hood above to remove the fumes from the air.
- Consider using an air purifier like the Germ Guardian above in your bedroom, as this will cut down on the problems with air quality in the bedrooms.
- If you have pets, keep them out of the bedrooms to reduce air quality issues in the bedrooms.
- If you use any scents, air fresheners in the home, read the labels. Anything that isn't 100% natural and has the word "fragrance" on the back is potentially problematic. If you can't figure out when is in it, don't inhale it. If you smell it, you're inhaling it. Fresh cut flowers, dried flowers, all natural air fresheners with the actual plant and media like alcohol are probably safe, but be weary of many of the rest.

How can I curb my behaviors to reduce risk of indoor pollution exposure?

Start with the following questions and jot down a few responses:

1. What do you smell in your home? Cooking oil/grease? Synthetic fragrances? Smoke?

    _____

    _____

    _____

    _____

2. Of those things listed above, what could you reduce?

    _____

    _____

    _____

    _____

3. If you can not reduce the things above, what could you do to reduce the impact?

    _____

    _____

_____

_____

4. What ways can you advocate for clean air for friends and families?

_____

_____

_____

Non-Stick Surfaces and Waterproofing Spray Worksheet

What is this?

You answered that you may be using non-stick surfaces on your pots and pans or use of waterproofing spray on your clothing.

Why do we care?

Non-stick surfaces and waterproofing spray have been associated with cancer.

Your homework, if you are not aware of this is to watch "The Devil We Know." It's a documentary on non-stick surfaces. It is available on Netflix, but can be purchased in multiple places over the web, including Amazon Prime and Apple Movies.

This documentary is epic. It will change the way you think about non-stick surfaces forever.

---

[3] "Get the Facts." The Devil We Know Documentary. https://thedevilweknow.com/get-the-facts/ Accessed May 21st, 2019.

[4] Teflon and Perfluorooctanoic Acid (PFOA). American Cancer Society. https://www.cancer.org/cancer/cancer-causes/teflon-and-perfluorooctanoic-acid-pfoa.html. Accessed May 22nd, 2019.

Here's a few of the statistics that are very disturbing. PFOA (Perfluorooctanoic acid) is a toxic chemical found in non-stick surfaces and is now found in 99% of Americans.[3]

Disease causes by water, air, and soil pollution are responsible for 9 million premature deaths annually-that's 16% of all global deaths.[1]

"The **International Agency for Research on Cancer (IARC)** is part of the World Health Organization (WHO). One of its goals is to identify causes of cancer. IARC has classified PFOA as "possibly carcinogenic to humans" (Group 2B), based on limited evidence in humans that it can cause testicular and kidney cancer, and limited evidence in lab animals."[4]

What can be done?

There is a lot of money invested in defending the use of non-stick surfaces and waterproofing spray: it's a multi-million industry. The question isn't if it's safe, it's how much is safe or isn't safe. We have a choice. We are exposed to many cancer-causing agents unknowingly already.

We can refuse to use any non-stick surfaces in our homes. We can educate friends, families and colleagues about the dangers. We can ask when we are eating out if the kitchens are using non-stick surfaces. If they are, we can ask if they can use alternatives.

We can refuse to use waterproof clothing used with PFAs and waterproofing sprays.

What can I do?

PFAa (polyfluoroalkyl substances) are found in many consumer products: non-stick cookware, food packaging, water proof clothing, stain-resistant carpeting, dental floss, etc.[1]

Studies have found that it takes 2-5 minutes on a stovetop to exceed temperatures at which non-stick surfaces overheat, emitting toxic particles and gases.[1]

Start by getting rid of all the non-stick surfaces in the house. This is not easy. You will find that they are present on top of griddles, waffle makers, pots/pans, even coffee pots, etc. Also many of the utensils used for cooking in the kitchen are made with non-stick surfaces.

Try and get rid of clothing that contains PFAs or waterproofing material.

Start with the following questions and jot down a few responses:

1. How often do I use nonstick surfaces?

_____

_____

_____

_____

_____

2. Why do I use nonstick surfaces?

_____

_____

_____

_____

_____

3. Are there times where I have used alternatives to nonstick surfaces? What alternatives are there?

_____

_____

_____

_____

_____

4. What can I do to reduce or completely eradicate my use of nonstick surfaces?

_____

_____

_____

_____

_____

Fragrances Worksheet

What is this?

You answered that you have regular exposures to fragrances. Fragrances are potentially harmful.

Why do we care?

Many of us use fragrances in our homes, on our bodies, in our care. These chemical scents use fragrance(s) which are not FDA approved for safety. They are protected by the US Patent Office, so we can't even determine what's in them. We are completely vulnerable to these chemicals, often breathing them in 700-100 times per hour (12-20 times per minute) all day long.

These scented products contain carcinogenic chemicals, lung irritants, phthalates and hormone disrupting chemicals.[5]

Carcinogenic chemicals are chemicals that cause cancer. We are often exposed to potentially carcinogenic chemicals. Creating anxiety about what we are all exposed to is not helpful. In today's world, we are unlikely to be able to reduce our risks of exposure to zero. But, we have taken the opposite approach and choose to simply "not worry about it."

Lung irritants cause a direct chemical irritation to the lungs. People with asthma experience bronchospasm or wheezing, chest tightness, and even respiratory distress. It's important to avoid lung irritants, particularly if you are hypersensitive, have allergies, asthma, emphysema, COPD, chronic bronchitis, or other lung disease.

Phthalate exposures are widespread in the U.S. population.[6] Exposure occurs from eating and drinking foods that have been in contact with

---

[5] Stink! https://stinkmovie.com/take-action/. Accessed May 26th, 2019.
[6] "Phthalates Factsheet."

containers and products containing phthalates, or breathing air containing phthalates.[2] They are generally thought to affect our reproductive system. In boys and men, they may lower testosterone. The EPA is conducting ongoing surveillance, but generally phthalates should be avoided. They are also used in plastics, raincoats, cosmetics, shampoos, air fresheners.

There is a catch-all term for hormone-disrupting chemicals which are chemicals which are thought to disrupt testosterone, feminizing men or reducing their testosterone. In addition, women may receive too much estrogen, leading to breast cancers, uterine cancers or other hormone-sensitive cancers.

What can be done?

Create fragrance-free zones at home. You have heard this often throughout the program, but fragrance has evidence that it is harmful. Why take the risk of harm?

Yes, the data is not definitive at this point, but it's starting to stack up. You don't want to be the person who finds out the hard way that you have developed cancer, because of fragrances. In addition, if you have children or grandchildren in the home you don't want to expose them to something that ends up causing cancer.

Your homework is to watch the documentary Stink. Learn more by checking out the website at https://stinkmovie.com. Check out the #StinkMovie to follow and learn more. This documentary will be somewhat alarming, but I think will be a helpful overview of the problem at hand.

What can I do?

https://www.cdc.gov/biomonitoring/Phthalates_FactSheet.html. Accessed May 28th, 2019.

Start by removing any products in the home that create artificial fragrance. If you have plug-ins or other fragrance devices, let's get rid of all those things first.

Then, look at your cleaning products. From dish soap to cleaning products for the kitchen and bathroom. Let's reduce all products in the home that have added fragrance to them.

Then, let's look at cosmetics, shampoo, soaps, detergents in the bathroom to determine where there are potential fragrance exposures. Find those products and eliminate them.

There are potential replacements, like all natural perfumes, essential oils, which use only alcohol and the product containing scent. We much prefer these products. They will keep things smelling nice, without the harm delineated above.

Start with the following questions and jot down a few responses:

1. How often do I use fragrances? Where do I use fragrances?

_____

_____

_____

_____

2. Why do I use fragrances?

_____

_____

_____

_____

3. Are there times when I have tried to use alternatives or been aware of these exposures? How can I increase my awareness to these exposures?

_____

_____

_____

_____

4. What can I do to reduce or completely eradicate my use of fragrances?

_____

_____

_____

_____

5-Sense Skip™

Toxins are virtually everywhere. You will often hear people say, you can't avoid toxins, they are everywhere. It's true that it can be tough, but toxins are literally killing us, causing cancer, heart disease, diabetes, amidst numerous other diseases. We must stand up to toxins in a way that's practical and easy to remember.

Doctor of Living has developed a daily strategy to help you avoid them called the **5-Sense Skip™**. If you can taste it, see it, touch it, smell it or hear it and it's toxic, skip it. One great thing about our bodies is we were created with 5 senses to enjoy life, but also as a form of defense. It's time we started to trust our bodies and started to beef up our defenses against toxins. Life is too short and too precious to trust things that are proven to cause disease or EVEN those things that aren't proven but suspected.

Making good toxin free choices is part of your **Health Improvement Action Plan™**. Here's how the **5-Sense Skip™** works:

Taste-
> ➤ If you taste unnatural products in food, stop eating them.
> ➤ If you taste chemicals in the water you are drinking, stop drinking and find fresh water.
> ➤ If you taste chemicals in the air you are breathing, have your air tested, turn off the chemical room scent, find an environment without pollution.

Sight-
> ➤ If you see smoke in the air, avoid it.
> ➤ If you see labels at the store on food you are looking to buy and ingredients you don't recognize, skip it.

- If the food at the store doesn't say organic AND you can afford the organic option, buy organic.
- If the food at the store says that it has GMOs, buy those that don't.
- If the food has any exposure to pesticides, do NOT eat them. There is no pesticide threshold I would consume and I wouldn't recommend it for you. No matter what the "safe threshold" it's not enough to keep your family safe.

Touch

- Clothing that you touch that has chemicals from dry cleaning or other chemicals that burn or irritate the skin should be removed from your skin.
- When you touch cleaning agents and you feel burning sensation, you should avoid them.
- When you touch greasy chemicals, be sure you know what's in them. Natural chemicals for skin lubrication or painful, cracked hands may be ok, but avoid unnatural, unidentifiable chemicals in skin care.

Smell

- If you smell burning meat or other animal products, you are probably being exposed to advanced glycation end products, which can cause cancer. Avoid areas with burning, grilling animal products.
- If you smell chemicals from exhaust of machinery, move to safe air.
- If you smell cleaning products in the air, plug-in scents in the home, inquire about their safety and if unknown, move to safety.
- If you smell gases or fumes from furniture, move to safety and avoid them.
- New homes are often tightly sealed, if there are smells in your home, move to safety.
- If you work somewhere with toxic smells, inquire about them, understand them. You have a right to know what you are breathing.

Sound

- Sound pollution has been shown to cause anxiety, heart disease amidst others. If you are constantly hearing sound pollution, consider a quieter place for reflection daily. Invest in noise cancelling headphones to give yourself a break from sound pollution.

➤ Ask ALL THE TIME about ingredients and chemicals. If you haven't heard of them, don't buy it, put in on or in your body.

Each day when you are out and about, consider the **5-Sense Skip™.** Let it guide your daily consumption and steer you to safety when chemicals and toxins are lurking. It's easy to remember your 5 senses and it's much better to skip out on things you aren't sure about and seek clarification.

There are many chemicals that are dangerous to us, but there are also dozens of responsible organizations, such as the Environmental Working group. If you are in doubt, check out their website https://www.ewg.org. They have a huge database of safe chemicals.

Good luck and be safe out there. Avoiding toxins isn't futile. It takes commitment and a new mentality of considering toxins in your daily life!

3-Part Cut Diet™

Stop Eating Meat. Stop Eating Dairy. Stop Eating Sugar.

According to Merriam-Webster's Dictionary, **diet** is defined as *"food and drink regularly provided or consumed."* It's (diet) origins are from the 13th century and it's original meaning in English was *"habitually taken food and drink."* There are numerous other definitions, particularly as it relates to losing weight and restricting food or drink. I like *"habitually taken food and drink,"* as to me this is what one's diet is and should be all about.

Most of us understand the word **diet** to be a temporary change in one's food and drink to achieve a desired outcome, such as weight loss. Personally, I have never understood the concept of a temporary change in what we eat or drink for a measured or unmeasured outcome. To me, this has no purpose, as temporarily changing one's diet for a desired outcome means that after this outcome is obtained, a person will go back to eating and drinking the way they did prior to the temporary change.

If a person desires weight loss or lifestyle changes, then why not change your lifestyle or diet completely, without any plan to ever go back to your old ways? If you plan to live healthier, then bravo! But, don't pretend to live better for a short time and then hop back on the previous unhealthy train. This is NOT sustainable.

Diets that preach quick weight loss often prey on your desire to find a healthier you, but quick promises lead to quick disappointment. At Doctor of Living, we believe in sustainable change that you can live with. The results are impressive and do take time, but it's well worth it!

If you are interested in changing your diet, then let's pick some changes that are simple, easy to remember and one's you can live with. Here are 3 changes everyone should make.

1) **Stop Eating Meat**

Meat is loaded with fat and all kinds of other bad things. According to caloriecount.com, a 3 oz (85 g) Beef Tenderloin has 247 calories, 155 from fat. 17.2 g of total fat. Saturated fat is 6.8 g, polyunsaturated fat 0.7 g, and monounsaturated fat 7.1 g. It is 73 mg of cholesterol. Let's compare that with Tofu (1/2 cup or 126 g) . According to caloriecount.com, There are 88 calories in Tofu. Total Fat is 5.3 grams and saturated fat is 1.1 gram. Polyunsaturated fat is 2.3 g and monounsaturated fat is 1.5 g. There is no cholesterol in Tofu.

FOOD	CALORIES	FAT CAL	TOTAL FAT	SAT. FAT	POLYUN	MONO	CHOLEST
BEEF TENDER-LOIN (3 OUNCES)	247	155	17.2	6.8	0.7	7.1	73
TOFU (1/2 CUP)	88		5.3	1.1	2.3	1.5	0
BEEF TENDER-LOIN (9 OUNCES)	741			20.4			219

I don't know about you, but I rarely see any tenderloin of 3 oz served. I think that 6-9 oz is more common. At the Outback Restaurant (http://outback.com/), you have the option of 6 or 9 oz filet mignon, but not 3 oz. So double or even triple the amount of fat. That's 34.4 or even 41.8 g overall of fat. In a 9 oz tenderloin, you are looking at 20.4 grams of unsaturated fat and 219 mg of cholesterol vs a serving of tofu has no cholesterol and 3 servings would be 15.9 overall grams of fat and 3.3 of saturated fat. That's a big difference! Nobody eats meat for fat though, right…it's all about the protein???

What about the protein then? Per howmuchprotein.com, Soy beans have 35.9g of protein per 100 grams (375 kcal) of soy beans vs 20.9 g in 100g (155 kcal) of beef. Soy beans contain all 8 essential amino acids. Of course, there's no fat in soy beans.

FOOD	PROTEIN	CONTAINS ALL 8 ESSENTIAL AMINO ACIDS?
SOY BEANS	35.9g	Yes
BEEF	20.9g	Yes

If you switched from beef to soy beans, you would add protein, cut fat and cholesterol.

Maybe you feel like this is part of your habitual food and that's it's unlikely that you'll be able to change. Let's take a look at the beef industry statistics from beefusa.org. The beef industry is an $88.25 billion industry. There were 92 million head of cattle and calves on Jan 1, 2016 in the US. US commercial slaughter was 28.74 million head in 2015. Total beef production was 23.69 billion pounds at $6.29/lb for choice beef. You might want to think hard about your habitual consumption of beef, because your habit may very well be determined by the popularity of beef consumption and the marketing that goes with a $88 billion industry. "Beef...it's what's for dinner" may have influenced your habits more than you think. The lobbyist power in Washington DC from the Beef Industry may also be influencing the USDA recommendations for meat in our diets and thereby influencing your preferences. Don't be an advertising victim. Make choices based on your desired health, rather than someone's desire to sell you something.

Per the World Health Organization, there is Group 2A evidence that red meat, defined as beef veal, pork, lamb, mutton, horse and goat, is **carcinogenic.** The strongest relationship is between red meat and colorectal cancer, but also evidence that it could cause pancreatic cancer and prostate cancer. This is a very contentious issue, as you might imagine and with the previously mentioned data on the meat industry, you understand that there are billions of dollars at stake. If there's a question of health, don't be a lab rat and wait for something to happen to you. Avoid it!

2) **Stop Eating Dairy**

Dairy is loaded with fat, which causes us to get fat and fills our vessels with cholesterol, increasing risk of heart disease and stroke. In addition, it's loaded with hormones, which have been associated with several types of cancers, including prostate, breast, and other hormone sensitive cancers.

There are numerous foods that will get calcium in our diet, without the risks of dairy. Low oxalate foods, like broccoli, bok choy, kale, Napa cabbage, watercress, mustard and turnip greens.

Many Americans are vitamin D deficient, even when consuming dairy. Taking a daily multivitamin, which includes Vitamin D may be helpful. Take to your doctor first, but this is another way to ensure adequate Vitamin D.

The bottom line with dairy is that it's not healthy and there are better alternatives with plants.

3) **Stop Eating Foods with Sugar and Refined Flour.**

Sugar can include fruit although whole fruit includes fiber as well and therefore has nutritional value. Processed sugar like white sugar, brown sugar, honey, agave, and coconut sugar are all nutrient lacking sugar that should be avoided.

We don't think about white bread, white pasta, refined flour as being the equivalent to sugar, but our bodies see it that way. Try and cut out all consumption of refined flour products, which include any breads, pasta, etc. created with white flour. Whole grain breads and past are ok, but should be 100% whole grain.

Sugar is added into everything. The bottom line for the program is that if it has added sugar, honey, syrup, corn syrup or any other sweetener, let's cut it out.

162

Spiritual Letters

Description:

*This is an **optional** activity, as some people may feel uncomfortable with God. The Well90 Program incorporates spiritual health into overall emotional and physical health. Our spirituality is the basis by which we see and interact with the World. Below you will find a number of different themes, all related to your spiritual health. If you are using this workbook with the Well90 Program, the themes will be prioritized for you. You can use them independently, as well.*

Each theme will call upon you to write a letter. Some letters, will be directly to God and others towards other people. Feel free to pull out a journal, buy a new notebook or refurbish an old one. You can also use loose paper, stationary or whatever you are comfortable with. You can even type them up and save them on your desktop.

Instructions:

This workbook is designed for you and you alone. You are free to share your letters with trusted others, but your answers and thoughts will likely be more genuine if you keep them private. Recognize that the letters may contain sensitive information that you may not want anyone to find. Keep them safe!

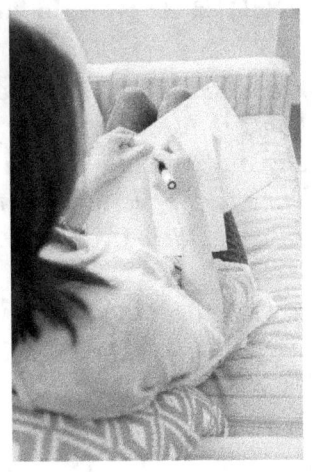

Each theme will have a new spiritual devotion to reflect upon. You will be challenged to write a letter specific to that theme.

We will explore your past, present and future. As you do so, you may experience joy and comfort, pain and remorse, or even fear. It is natural to feel these emotions. Just as when you meditate, try to experience these emotions without any judgment. You are not alone in having many emotions about your spiritual well-being. It is healthy to experience all of these emotions, without judging them.

Directions: *Sit down in a quiet spot each day. Find a clean journal, notebook or even blank piece of paper. Close the door to the room, if you can. Close your eyes. Take a few deep breaths and feel God's presence in your life.*

Theme 1: How do you communicate with God?

In the morning, when you wake up, look at your day. What are the issues that you face in the day? What are the challenges? Start off with an open letter to God about your concerns. Invite help into your life. Ask for specific things. Offer thanks for specific things.

Do this each day for one week, taking off Sunday to reflect on what you have written.

Theme 2: How do you feel God's presence?

Write this letter to God, telling God where you feel God's presence. You should think about where you feel God's presence? At work? At home? At a religious institution? In a relationship? Acknowledge God's presence or the divine in your letter. Where else might you consider looking for God's presence during your day.

Do this each day for one week, taking off Sunday to reflect on what you have written.

Theme 3: We often compartmentalize our lives. This is where God lives and this is where I am secular. How do you reunify God with your every moment?

Write this letter to God. Acknowledge places, times, and relationships where you compartmentalize God. This may be intended to avoid offending anyone or out of necessity at work. Acknowledge these places, times and situations in your letters. In addition, seek out opportunities to reunify God in every situation. Tell God when and where you intend to reunify.

Do this each day for one week, taking off Sunday to reflect on what you have written.

Theme 4: Do you have peace in your relationship with God/Divine?

Write this letter to God. Acknowledge past hurt with God, religion in your letter. Find opportunities to achieve peace with God. Look for opportunities to forgive others and God. Define where you would like to end up in your relationship with God.

Do this each day for one week, taking off Sunday to reflect on what you have written.

Theme 5: What is your desired relationship with God/Divine?

Write this letter to God. What would the optimal relationship with God look like? How will you communicate going forward? How frequently? How will you remind yourself of God's presence? How will you reunify God into your life? How will you forgive and keep forgiveness in your heart, when you feel hurt or wronged by God?

Do this each day for one week, taking off Sunday to reflect on what you have written.

Theme 6: Do you feel love for people you don't know?

Write a letter to someone you have never met. Choose a picture in a newspaper, on TV. Someone you don't know at all. You shouldn't even really know their story. Write them a love letter. Not a mushy love letter, but a letter that expresses your genuine love and concern for them. You don't need to send it. Identify all the ways in which you love them. Give specifics and express thanks for both the things you love about that person, as well as the love itself.

Do this each day for one week, taking off Sunday to reflect on what you have written.

Theme 7: **Do you feel love for those in the community or someone you might know?**

Write a love letter to someone in your community who did something you disliked. This could be a clerk at a store, someone who cheated you. This letter also doesn't need to be sent. This will be very challenging. Humanity falls short of meeting our expectations, but also falls short of God's expectations. As you think about love, think about why you might have challenges trying to loving someone you dislike.

Do this each day for one week, taking off Sunday to reflect on what you have written.

Theme 8: **Do you feel love for those in a close-knit relationship?**

Write a letter to someone that you don't love currently, but know that you should. This should be someone you are supposed to have a close-knit relationship with. This may be more difficult. It may be easier to think about someone who you feel like you should love more or love better than you do. Either way, write them a love letter. Again, you don't need to send it. Be honest about your lack of love or desire to have greater love and tell them the truth. Identify ways you could love them more.

Do this each day for one week, taking off Sunday to reflect on what you have written.

Theme 9: **Do you feel love for yourself?**

Sometimes our love we experience for ourselves is the most challenging of all. Think about all of the wonderful things that you love about yourself. No qualifiers. No filters. This is your moment to write it all down and let yourself know just how amazing you are! Be specific. List everything out and, most importantly, define why you feel the way you do.

Do this each day for one week, taking off Sunday to reflect on what you have written.

Theme 10: **Are you aware of yourself?**

Self-awareness is an important part about connecting with the World, as well as ourselves. Write a letter to yourself about how you see yourself. If you were to walk into a room of perfect strangers, how would they describe you? How would an old friend describe you? How would he or she describe you? Write a new letter to yourself about how you want to be seen not only to friends, but to World you don't know? Where are the gaps? Where are the opportunities to reinvent yourself to the World?

Do this each day for one week, taking off Sunday to reflect on what you have written.

Theme 11: **Do you feel at peace?**
Peace is defined by Wikipedia as "freedom from disturbance; tranquility."

Write a letter to someone specific in the community or the community at large that you don't know. Our sense of peace has a lot to do with our view of our communities. Identify times, places and situations where you found true peace in your community. Maybe at a community gathering or in the park. Express thanks and gratitude for these moments to those in your community you may not know now, but could know someday. Identify

167

opportunities where you could find peace in the future. Identify hurdles or obstacles that might make peace difficult during at times. Identify ways that can help you persevere and develop peace in new situations.

Do this each day for one week, taking off Sunday to reflect on what you have written.

Theme 12: **What brings you joy?**

Joy isn't the same as peace. Joy is defined by Wikipedia as "a feeling of great pleasure and happiness."

Joy gives our lives meaning. With joy, comes desire to experience connections. Often, we get busy during the weeks, months and years. We get caught up in tasks, outcomes, materialism. We forget about joy. Think about the last time you experienced joy in a relationship.

Let's recall the last time you experienced joy in a specific relationship. Write a "Thank You" note the person you have a close- knit relationship with for the joy you experienced with them. While writing your "thank you" recall the specific reasons why you felt joyful. Ask for help in recognizing future joyful moments.

Do this each day for one week, taking off Sunday to reflect on what you have written.

Theme 13: **Who do you respect?**

We best form healthy connections, when we have self-respect. When we have self-respect, we are true to ourselves. Write a letter to yourself recalling a time, when you struggled to show respect for yourself. Maybe it was a lapse in judgment or something you regret. Do you think it's possible to withhold respect for yourself, while maintaining respect for God? Are there opportunities in your life where you could offer greater respect to yourself and others?

Do this each day for one week, taking off Sunday to reflect on what you have written.

Theme 14: **What does your life mean to you?**

Forgiveness has everything to do with the meaning we place to our existence. Identify what you view as the meaning of your life. What is your purpose? Who do you serve? What difference do you make each day in your existence?

Every one of us falls short of our expectations. Where have you fallen short? What opportunities are there to improve? In what ways, can you forgive yourself for not living up to your life's purpose?

Do this each day for one week, taking off Sunday to reflect on what you have written.

Theme 15: **Are you expressing kindness in a proud way?**

Part of being able to forgive someone in your community, is an act of kindness. During this week, you will write about kindness. Wikipedia defines kindness as "the quality of being friendly, generous, and considerate" All of us have been kind and all of us have been unkind. Address your letters to your community this week, expressing your forgiveness for a time when someone or somebody did something to wrong you. Each day offer one example of a time you were wronged, but did not give forgiveness. Then, offer an example of when you did offer forgiveness and were kind to yourself and someone else.

Ask for help in being present in the moment when kindness is required. Ask God to help you become kinder towards others.

Do this each day for one week, taking off Sunday to reflect on what you have written.

Theme 16: **Are you forgiving those you love?**

Many of us are unaware that we are withholding forgiveness, even to those we love dearly. You can still love someone, without forgiving them. It's complicated right! We all know this, but it's time to forgive the hurt.

Write a letter to someone you love dearly, but have been unable to forgive to this point. This person doesn't even have to be living. The most important part is that the letter offers forgiveness, even if the person never solicited it. In some cases, they may have never been aware that you were hurt. That's ok too. Again, be sure that letter is written directly to this person.

Do this each day for one week, taking off Sunday to reflect on what you have written.

Theme 17: **Are you forgiving yourself for your past?**

It is difficult to forgive others, when we are not forgiving ourselves. None of us are perfect. Because of this, it's time to forgive ourselves for past hurt. Things we did that we regret. Things that betrayed our values or integrity. We have all done things that we need forgiveness for and we are withholding forgiveness.

Write a letter to yourself detailing what you want forgiveness for. Keep this letter locked up or delete or destroy it quickly. Forgive yourself for the pain. This will help to heal other relationships too.

Do this each day for one week, taking off Sunday to reflect on what you have written.